THE SKINNY TASTE MEAL PREP

Healthy Recipes with 7 Ingredients or Fewer

Adam C.

ISBN: 9798871119440

DEDICATION

This book is dedicated to all my Readers

CONTENTS

Chapter 1: Introduction

Thank you for visiting "The Skinny Taste Meal Prep: Healthy Recipes with 7 Ingredients or Fewer." This chapter serves as an introduction to the world of mindful meal preparation. It covers the fundamentals of Skinny Taste Meal Prep, the many advantages of adopting this style of cooking, and useful advice on how to make meal planning both efficient and healthful.

1.1 About Skinny Taste Meal Prep

1. A Culinary Philosophy: More than just a cookbook, Skinny Taste Meal Prep is a cooking philosophy that emphasizes flavor, health, and simplicity. The fundamental focus of Skinny Taste Meal Prep is on the skill of preparing scrumptious and wholesome meals using the fewest possible ingredients. The emphasis is on quality, making sure that every food is enjoyable to taste as well as simple to prepare.

2. The Skinny Taste Legacy: Started by popular food blogger and author Gina Homolka, Skinny Taste has grown to be a reputable brand in the realm of tasty and nutritious dishes. Gina, who has a love for cooking nutritious food that is also tasty, has developed a community of home cooks who are willing to make healthy decisions without sacrificing flavor.

3. Why Meal Prep Matters: Choosing to prepare your meals in advance can change your perspective on food and is more than just a fad. You can control what goes into your meals, how much you eat, and ultimately, your health, if you plan and prepare them ahead of time. This idea is expanded upon by Skinny Taste Meal Prep, which makes it pleasurable and approachable for people leading hectic lives.

1.2 Benefits of Meal Prep

1. Time-Saving Magic: The substantial time savings that come with establishing a meal prep routine are among its main benefits. It might be difficult to find the time to prepare healthful meals every day in our hectic life. This process is made easier with Skinny Taste Meal Prep, which lets you set out a few hours per week to make meals that you can eat all week long.

2. Health at the Core: Fundamentally, health is achieved through thoughtful meal preparation, which encourages better eating practices. You can make deliberate decisions that support your dietary objectives by managing the ingredients and amount sizes. With the help of Skinny Taste Meal Prep recipes, you can easily maintain a healthy and balanced diet by maximizing nutritional content and minimizing needless additives.

3. Financial Wellness: Meal preparation can support financial wellbeing in addition to time savings and health promotion. Making strategic grocery purchases when you plan your meals ahead of time lowers the chance of making expensive and impulsive eating choices. You may make economic decisions with Skinny Taste Meal Prep without compromising on nutrition or taste.

4. Reduced Stress: Bid farewell to the everyday strain of figuring out what to make for supper or stressing over last-minute food possibilities. You'll feel lighter and more in control of your weekly meals when you follow Skinny Taste Meal Prep's well-thought-out schedule. This method helps you feel less stressed and more accomplished because you are able to feed your family and yourself healthful meals on a regular basis.

1.3 Tips for Efficient Meal Planning

1. Mastering the Basics: Learning the fundamentals is the first step towards effective meal planning. Make a weekly meal plan that includes your breakfasts, lunches, dinners, and snacks to get started. Be mindful of your calendar, taking into account hectic days, possible out-of-town eating occasions, and social gatherings.

2. Diverse and Balanced: Just as diversity adds flavor to life, so too should your meals. Make sure the meals in your meal plan are varied; incorporate a variety of fruits, vegetables, whole grains, and meats. This guarantees that you get a wide variety of nutrients and also adds interest to your meals.

3. Strategic Ingredient Use: The key to the success of Skinny Taste Meal Prep is the thoughtful application of ingredients. Accept the idea of using fewer ingredients without sacrificing flavor. To give your weekly menu coherence, select adaptable foods that may be used in several meals during the week.

4. Batch Cooking Techniques: Make the most of your time and energy by using strategies for batch cooking. Make bigger batches of basic components so they can be used as the foundation for several recipes. As you mix and match ingredients, this not only simplifies the cooking procedure but also permits creative culinary expression.

5. Invest in Quality Storage: Without appropriate storage options, effective meal planning is inadequate. Invest in high-quality containers to preserve the flavor and freshness of your food. For added convenience, think about dividing meals into individual portions for grab-and-go options. Proper storage guarantees that your culinary endeavors yield enduring and delectable outcomes.

Remember these guidelines as you start your Skinny Taste Meal Prep journey. This cookbook is a manual for changing the way you feel about eating, not just a list of recipes. You may experience the satisfaction of providing wholesome, delectable meals for your family and yourself by practicing mindful planning, deliberate ingredient selection, and a dedication to simplicity. Prepare to welcome a new approach to cooking and eating that reflects the delight of a well-prepared meal and is in line with your wellness objectives.

Chapter 2: Kitchen Essentials

A variety of utensils and basic ingredients are the cornerstones of any well-prepared kitchen and serve as the basis for tasty and nutritious meals. We explore the key components in this chapter that make Skinny Taste Meal Prep enjoyable to use as well as approachable. Let's examine the essentials of a well-stocked and effective kitchen, from essential appliances that speed up your cooking to basic ingredients that serve as the foundation of our meals.

2.1 Must-Have Tools

1. Cutting Boards: Commence your culinary exploration with a robust collection of chopping boards. To avoid cross-contamination, use separate cutting boards for fruits, vegetables, and meats. This improves the organization of your prep work and guarantees the safety of the food.

2. Chef's Knife: The workhorse of the kitchen is an excellent chef's knife. Purchase a sturdy, well-balanced knife that fits well in your hand. This multipurpose implement will accompany you while you chop, slice, and dice a range of items.

3. Mixing Bowls: For both preparation and serving, a collection of mixing bowls in different sizes is essential. Choose bowls with sturdy construction that can tolerate vigorous mixing and stirring. Having a variety enables you to work on several aspects of a recipe at once.

4. Measuring Tools: Accuracy is essential in cooking, particularly when using recipes that call for portion management. To ensure precise ingredient measurements, get measuring spoons and cups. This is especially important if you are working with seven ingredients or less, as each one is essential to the finished product.

5. Non-Stick Skillet: A dependable non-stick pan is an indispensable tool in the kitchen, ideal for stir-frying, sear-frying, and sautéing for effortless clean up, pick a skillet with a non-stick surface and a robust build. With little effort, you can make a variety of Skinny Taste Meal Prep dishes with this adaptable pan.

6. Baking Sheets and Pans: A good set of baking sheets and pans is essential whether you're roasting veggies or making a sheet pan supper. To guarantee that your food cooks evenly, look for products with even heat distribution. This is especially crucial for making well-balanced flavors with little ingredients.

7. Food Processor or Blender: A food processor or blender is quite helpful for recipes that call for smooth sauces, dips, or finely chopped ingredients. With the help of these instruments, you can give your Skinny Taste Meal Prep recipes more depth by transforming simple foods into rich, savory components.

8. Storage Containers: Proper storage is essential for effective food preparation, which goes beyond cooking. Purchase a range of storage containers, ranging in size from tiny to large, to suit varying serving sizes. To keep your prepped meals as fresh as possible, use freezer-safe and airtight container selections.

9. Slow Cooker or Instant Pot: These appliances can be lifesavers on days when time is at a premium. With the help of these gadgets, you can simply set and forget as delectable meals simmer and become more complex with less manual labor.

10. Spiralizer: If you want to give your dishes a creative flair, think about include a spiralizer in your arsenal. This useful tool turns veggies into shapes resembling noodles, providing a low-carb substitute for regular spaghetti. It's a great way to add extra veggies to your meals without sacrificing flavor or satisfaction.

2.2 Staple Ingredients

1. Lean Proteins: A key component of Skinny Taste Meal Prep is constructing a meal around a lean source of protein. Keep foods like fish, poultry breast, lean ground turkey, and plant-based proteins like lentils or tofu in your kitchen. The foundation of a good and well-balanced meal is these proteins.

2. Whole Grains: Including whole grains in your meals gives them more fiber and nutrients. Stock your cupboard with a range of grains, such as quinoa, brown rice, farro, and oats. These adaptable essentials provide a healthy foundation for your dishes and may be used as the basis for many Skinny Taste Meal Prep recipes.

3. Fresh Vegetables: A rainbow of fresh veggies adds a multitude of vitamins and minerals to your meals while also improving their aesthetic appeal. Stock up on essentials such as tomatoes, bell peppers, spinach, broccoli, and carrots. These vegetables offer taste and nutrients to a variety of meals that may be made with ease.

4. Flavorful Herbs and Spices: Adding flavor to your food without gaining extra calories is all thanks to herbs and spices. Add paprika, cumin, onion powder, garlic powder, and a variety of herbs including rosemary, thyme, and basil to your spice rack. You can maintain the flavor and excitement of your meals by experimenting with different combinations.

5. Healthy Fats: To give your meals depth and fullness, include sources of healthy fats. Nuts, seeds, avocado, and olive oil are all fantastic options. Your Skinny Taste Meal Prep dishes will taste great and filling because these fats not only improve the flavor of your food but also help you feel fuller.

6. Low-Sodium Broths and Stocks: Stock your pantry with low-sodium broths and stocks for an instant taste boost. These adaptable components add depth and richness to your dishes without adding too much salt when used as a foundation for soups, stews, and sauces.

7. Greek Yogurt: This adaptable ingredient works well in savory as well as sweet recipes. It can be used in sweets as well as dips and sauces to give them a creamy texture and base for dressings. If you want to keep your meals light and health-conscious, go for plain, non-fat Greek yogurt.

8. Citrus Fruits: Meals can be greatly enhanced by the vivid and zesty flavors of citrus fruits like lemons and limes. Store these fruits for their juice and zest, which you can use to infuse a number of meals with a burst of flavor and acidity.

9. Dijon Mustard: Low in calories and high in flavor, Dijon mustard is a condiment. This adaptable ingredient may be used to marinades, dressings, and sauces, giving your Skinny Taste Meal Prep recipes a tangy and slightly spicy touch.

10. Honey or Maple Syrup: Stock your cupboard with either of these for a hint of natural sweetness. As a healthier substitute for processed sugars, these natural sweeteners can be used sparingly to balance flavors in both savory and sweet recipes.

Not only are you cooking meals when you stock your kitchen with these essential tools and basic supplies, but you're also laying the groundwork for a way of life that values delectable, healthful food. The foundation of Skinny Taste Meal Prep is the harmony of these tools and ingredients, which makes it a useful and pleasurable method for preparing meals that feed the body and the soul. We'll apply these fundamentals to a range of meals in the next chapters that highlight the simplicity and freshness of the Skinny Taste Meal Prep concept. Prepare to turn your kitchen into a center of inventive cooking and healthful food.

Chapter 3: 7-Ingredient Magic

Simplicity is king in the magical world of Skinny Taste Meal Prep. This chapter reveals the secret to cooking nutritious and delectable meals using only seven ingredients or less. You'll learn that making delectable and healthful meals can be simple and enjoyable as we examine the power of simplicity, dive into the art of selecting the proper ingredients, and hone the skill of wise replacements.

3.1 Exploring the Power of Simplicity

1. Embracing Minimalism: The secret to the success of Skinny Taste Meal Prep is its dedication to simplicity in a world where options and complexity may be overwhelming. The idea behind utilizing seven ingredients or fewer each recipe is to fully embrace the essence of each component, not to impose any restrictions. By concentrating on a small number of ingredients, we bring out the best in each one, letting their flavors come through and harmonize on the tongue.

2. Enhancing Flavor, Minimizing Complexity: Beyond being simple to prepare, simplicity has a direct impact on each dish's taste intensity. Reducing the quantity of ingredients encourages us to choose and combine them with more intention. Each ingredient is selected not just for its nutritional content but also for its capacity to improve the recipe's overall flavor profile. Meals prepared with this deliberate approach are not only delicious but also carefully thought out.

3. Streamlining the Cooking Process: Ease in the ingredients themselves inevitably leads to ease in the cooking method. Recipes from Skinny Taste Meal Prep are meant to be accessible to home chefs of all experience levels. Reducing the amount of steps and cooking time by reducing the ingredient list makes these recipes more manageable for time-pressed people looking to get healthy meals without compromising on taste.

4. Creating Culinary Harmony: The art of cooking harmoniously is where simplicity truly shines. Every component in the meal serves a distinct function. All the components work together to create a well-rounded and fulfilling dinner, from the main protein to the subtle herbs and spices. Recipes for Skinny Taste Meal Prep are proof that cooking simply doesn't have to sacrifice flavor rather, it should honor each flavor's inherent purity.

3.2 Choosing the Right Ingredients

1. Quality over Quantity: The meticulous selection of premium ingredients lays the groundwork for the enchantment of the seven ingredients. When you are working with fewer ingredients, each one becomes more significant. For maximum flavor and nutrition in every bite, use lean proteins, healthy grains, and seasonal, fresh produce.

2. Building Flavor Layers: Though the ingredient list may be short, Skinny Taste Meal Prep meals are designed to be anything from boring. The secret is to combine ingredients carefully so that layers of flavor are created. Think about the harmony of complimentary flavors, the contrast of textures, and the interaction of sweet and savory. Making dish combinations that work well together results in a dish that is interesting and delicious.

3. Strategic Use of Condiments: Condiments have the power to take a dish from good to extraordinary; they might be its unsung heroes. With the help of condiments like citrus liquids, balsamic vinegar, and Dijon mustard, Skinny Taste Meal Prep may enhance flavor and complexity without packing on the ingredients. These condiments improve the overall flavor profile by adding a punch of acidity and flavor.

4. Incorporating Fresh Herbs: A hidden weapon in the realm of seven-ingredient magic is fresh plants. A little chopped parsley, cilantro, or basil can make a plain dish taste amazing. Fresh herbs add a burst of freshness that improves and balances the other ingredients with their brightness and aroma.

5. Balancing Textures: An important but sometimes disregarded component of a fulfilling meal is texture. The dishes in Skinny Taste Meal Prep pay close attention to the harmony of textures to guarantee a satisfying meal. Every texture in the dish be it the flakiness of the fish, the crunch of the roasted almonds, or the tenderness of the sautéed vegetables contributes to its overall appeal.

6. Mindful Use of Fats: Including heart-healthy fats in your meal prep, such as those found in nuts, avocados, and olive oil, is a wise decision. These fats improve satiety in addition to adding to the dish's flavor and richness. When fats are used carefully, meals become both gratifying and nutrient-dense, keeping you full and energized.

3.3 Smart Substitutions

1. Flexibility in the Kitchen: Skinny Taste Meal Prep's versatility is what makes it so wonderful. Although recipes call for seven ingredients or less, there is plenty of leeway for clever substitutions based on dietary restrictions, personal tastes, or item availability. Making these recipes your own is made possible by mastering the skill of clever substitutions.

2. Protein Variations: Please feel free to experiment with other protein sources in accordance with your dietary needs. If a dish asks for chicken, think about using turkey, tofu, or lentils in it's instead. The secret is to select proteins that preserve the flavor of the dish while still meeting your dietary needs and tastes.

3. Vegetable Swaps: You can quickly alter a dish's vegetable component according to what's in season or easily accessible in your kitchen. If a recipe calls for broccoli and you happen to have cauliflower on hand, feel free to substitute it. Replace some of your veggies with different ones to provide variety to your meals without throwing off the overall balance.

4. Grain Choices: A lot of the Skinny Taste Meal Prep recipes have a nourishing base made of whole grains. Depending on your dietary requirements or preferences, try quinoa, brown rice, or farro among other grains. Selecting grains that provide the right texture and nutritional value without sacrificing the recipe's simplicity is crucial.

5. Adapting for Dietary Restrictions: The philosophy behind Skinny Taste Meal Prep is that each person has different dietary demands. Feel free to modify the recipes to suit your preferences or dietary needs. The recipes are made to fit a range of dietary needs, whether it's switching to dairy-free or gluten-free grains or modifying the seasoning to your preference.

6. Exploring Flavor Variations: Once you get the basic recipe down pat, feel free to experiment with different flavors. Try experimenting with different herbs, spices, or sauces to give a tried-and-true recipe a fresh take. The ingredient list's simplicity allows you to be creative and modify the recipes to fit your changing palate.

7. Portion Adjustments: One of the best things about Skinny Taste Meal Prep is that it lets you customize portions to suit your needs. The recipes offer flexibility to meet your individual nutritional objectives, whether you're wanting to minimize carbs, up the protein content, or change the serving size overall.

Remember that the purpose of Skinny Taste Meal Prep is to celebrate the joy of cooking and fuel your body with healthful, flavorful meals not to follow strict rules as you set out on the adventure of 7-ingredient magic. A delicious and approachable culinary experience is produced by combining the forces of simplicity, expert product selection, and astute substitution. We'll put these ideas into practice and explore a range of meals in the upcoming chapters, showcasing the simplicity and vibrancy of Skinny Taste Meal Prep's magic. Prepare to turn your kitchen into a creative and nourishing paradise, one tasty, simple recipe at a time.

Chapter 4: Breakfast Bliss

Within the context of Skinny Taste Meal Prep, breakfast is a celebration of flavors, textures, and nutrients in addition to being the most significant meal of the day. This chapter takes you on a journey into Breakfast Bliss, where we look at nourishing and speedy morning options that will set the stage for a vibrant and energetic day. Prepare to make breakfast a symphony of flavor and health, ranging from the ease of overnight oats to a range of morning treats with seven ingredients or less.

4. Quick and Nutritious Morning Options

1. Morning Rituals: Mornings frequently determine the overall tone of the day. Skinny Taste Meal Prep is aware of the need for breakfast options that are high in nutrients and easy to make, without sacrificing taste. In order to guarantee that you begin your day on a healthful note, these dishes are made to seamlessly integrate into your morning routines.

2. Balanced Breakfasts: A nutritious breakfast is essential for maintaining focus and energy levels throughout the day.

Breakfast recipes from Skinny Taste Meal Prep offer the ideal ratio of healthy fats, carbohydrates, and proteins. There's a tasty and healthy selection to fit your tastes, whether you enjoy savory or sweet breakfasts.

3. Efficiency in Execution: Mornings might be busy, so there's not always time for fancy cooking. Breakfasts from Skinny Taste Meal Prep are designed to be as efficient as possible. These dishes, which call for seven items or less, let you quickly prepare a healthy breakfast without compromising time. Making mornings stress-free and nutrient-rich is the aim.

4. Customization for Variety: You can never have too much variety in life, especially when it comes to breakfast. Breakfast recipes from Skinny Taste Meal Prep provide a blank canvas for personalization. Try varying the fruits, nuts, and seeds in your breakfast dishes to give them a unique flavor. The recipes' simplicity makes them an adaptable base for a wide range of taste combinations.

4.2 Overnight Oats and More

1. The Magic of Overnight Oats: The secret to Breakfast Bliss is overnight oat magic. The spirit of Skinny Taste Meal Prep is embodied in this adaptable and quick recipe. When rolled oats are combined with a few essential ingredients, overnight oats become a tasty, creamy meal that comes together quickly in the morning.

2. Basic Overnight Oats Formula: It's easy to customize your own batch of overnight oats by just using a basic formula. Mix together rolled oats, liquid (such milk or a dairy substitute), sweetener (like honey or maple syrup), and flavor enhancers (like cinnamon or vanilla essence). Add your preferred nuts, seeds, or fruits, and then let the oats soak in the fridge for the entire night. The outcome is a tasty, filling meal that can be eaten right out of the refrigerator.

3. Variations for Every Palate: The unlimited diversity that overnight oats offer is one of their many wonderful qualities. Tailor your oats to suit your dietary requirements, preferred flavors, and seasonal fruit availability. The possibilities are as varied as your taste senses, ranging from traditional pairings like banana and peanut butter to unique combos like mango and coconut.

4. Prep Once, Enjoy All Week: Beyond their ease of preparation, overnight oats are the best meal prep breakfast option. If you take a few minutes at the start of the week to prepare jars of overnight oats, you'll always have a quick breakfast available. Even on the busiest of days, you can start your mornings with a healthy and filling meal thanks to this time-saving technique.

5. Savory Breakfast Jars: Savory breakfast jars are a novel idea introduced by Skinny Taste Meal Prep, yet sweet overnight oats remain a beloved traditional. These savory variations offer a savory twist on the typical oat-based version with additions like quinoa, sautéed vegetables, and a hint of cheese or herbs. With a burst of savory flavor, savory breakfast jars are a lovely way to add some variety to your daily routine.

6. Egg Muffins for Protein Power: Egg muffins are one of the solutions provided by Skinny Taste Meal Prep for individuals who want a high-protein breakfast option. These portable, high-protein treats mix eggs with a range of ingredients, including cheese, veggies, and lean meats. If you bake them ahead of time, you'll have a satisfying and easy hot or cold breakfast choice.

7. Quick and Flavorful Smoothie Bowls: Another treasure from the Breakfast Bliss line is smoothie bowls. Tightly containing fruits, veggies, and a small amount of liquid, these bowls are a hydrating and high-nutrient choice for hectic mornings. Add some texture and taste to your smoothie bowl by adding toppings like granola, almonds, and seeds. The end result is a quick and aesthetically pleasing breakfast that tastes great.

8. Fluffy Pancakes with a Twist: Who says a nutritious breakfast regimen can't include pancakes? With seven ingredients or less, Skinny Taste Meal Prep transforms classic pancakes into a fluffy, nutrient-dense dish. Whole grains, fresh fruit, and a hint of sweetness transform these pancakes into a guilt-free treat that's perfect for special mornings.

9. Creative Parfait Combinations: In the realm of breakfasts for Skinny Taste Meal Prep, parfaits are a creative canvas. Greek yogurt, granola, fresh fruit, and a honey drizzle combine to create a visually pleasing parfait that is also a pleasant blend of flavors and textures. With so many combinations to choose from, parfaits can be customized to your exact preferences.

10. Portable Breakfast Bars for On-the-Go: For mornings when time is truly of the essence, Skinny Taste Meal Prep provides premade, portable breakfast bars. These bars are a quick and filling breakfast alternative since they include oats, almonds, seeds, and a hint of sweetness. If you prepare a large quantity at the start of the week, you'll always have a convenient and speedy breakfast on hand for hectic mornings.

As you go through Skinny Taste Meal Prep's Breakfast Bliss chapter, you'll see that mornings don't have to be complicated to be tasty and healthy. Every breakfast meal is designed to improve your morning experience, from the wonders of overnight oats to a range of morning treats made with seven ingredients or less. Savor the delight of beginning your day with a hearty and filling meal that sets the stage for a day full of energy and vitality as you set off on this culinary adventure. Prepare to change your morning routine, one delicious bite at a time.

Chapter 5: Lunch on the Go

Lunch is more than just a chance to recharge at lunchtime in the busy world of Skinny Taste Meal Prep; it's a chance to enjoy tasty, portable meals that keep you full and energized all day. This chapter is an exploration of Lunch on the Go, where we learn how to make salads, wraps, and other dishes with only seven items or less. Experience the delight of tasty, health-conscious lunches that easily fit into your hectic schedule.

5.1 Portable and Delicious Midday Meals

1. Lunchtime Challenges: Lunchtime meals present a unique set of difficulties because of time constraints, the demand for convenience, and the requirement for a filling yet quick meal. Skinny Taste Meal Prep steps up to the plate, providing a range of lunch options that are not only tasty and portable but also thoughtfully crafted to be as simple as possible. Even on the busiest days, you can make the most of your lunch break with these recipes.

2. The Importance of Balanced Lunches: The secret to sustaining energy and concentration into the afternoon is a well-balanced meal. Lunches made with Skinny Taste Meal Prep strike the ideal ratio of nutritious grains, fiber-rich veggies, healthy fats, and proteins. Together, these ingredients provide meals that satiate your palate and give you steady energy for the remainder of the day.

3. Efficiency in Preparation: The recipes for Lunch on the Go are designed with efficiency in mind. The idea is to maximize flavor and nutritional value while minimizing preparation time. These recipes make sure you have a tasty and nutritious lunch ready to go wherever your day takes you, whether you're packing it for work, school, or a day of errands.

4. Versatility for Different Lifestyles: Lunch on the Go recipes cater to the varied lives of those who are constantly on the go. These dishes offer flexibility in preparation and consumption, making them ideal for a variety of occasions, including a picnic in the park, a fast snack at your desk, or a carry-along for a day of discovery. The end product is a selection of sandwiches that fit well into your particular schedule.

5.2 Salads, Wraps, and Beyond

1. The Art of Wholesome Salads: With Skinny Taste Meal Prep, salads become more than just greens they become colorful, filling meals. Proteins, fresh veggies, and tasty dressings can all be combined to create a variety of colorful and savory salads. The secret is to select components that not only enhance the salad's nutritional profile but also produce a harmonious blend of flavors and sensations.

2. Protein-Packed Salad Bowls: Protein-rich salad bowls are available from Skinny Taste Meal Prep for people looking to increase the amount of protein in their midday meal. These salads add healthy meats, like grilled chicken, shrimp, or beans, to go beyond the conventional idea of just greens. The outcome is a filling and substantial salad that keeps you going.

3. Grain-Based Salad Innovations: Whole grains give salads more body and texture, which makes them a delicious addition to Lunch on the Go. Grain-based salad innovations, using brown rice, quinoa, or farro, are explored in Skinny Taste Meal Prep. With their harmonious proportions of fiber, minerals, and complex carbohydrates, these salads offer a healthy base.

4. Mason Jar Salad Mastery: Mason jar salads are a useful lunchtime option that also looks great. The technique of layering ingredients in a jar to keep them fresh until you're ready to eat is revealed in Skinny Taste Meal Prep. These salads are a tribute to the careful planning that goes into making a meal that's both attractive and delicious, from the dressing at the bottom to the leafy greens at the top.

5. Savory and Nutrient-Rich Wraps: A staple for lunch on-the-go, wraps provide a quick and adaptable way to savor a range of flavors. Savory and nutrient-dense wraps that go above and beyond are now available with Skinny Taste Meal Prep. These wraps are a portable treat that livens up your noon meal, whether they're loaded with lean meats, grilled veggies, or tasty spreads.

6. Creative and Flavorful Roll-Ups: Lunchtime gets a humorous touch with roll-ups. The technique of making inventive and tasty roll-ups with components like deli meats, cheese, and fresh veggies is explored in Skinny Taste Meal Prep. These little marvels are a wonderful way to sample a range of flavors in a single, portable package, in addition to being simple to make.

7. Nourishing and Satisfying Buddha Bowls: Buddha bowls, which combine a variety of ingredients into a nutritional and delicious meal, are a Lunch on the Go revelation. These bowls frequently include a blend of veggies, proteins, grains, and a tasty sauce. The Buddha bowl idea is embraced by Skinny Taste Meal Prep, which provides meals that highlight the elegance of simplicity and balance in a single bowl.

8. Portable Pita Pockets: Pita pockets are a lunchtime favorite because of how versatile and portable they are. Enjoyably portable and health-conscious pita pockets are now available from Skinny Taste Meal Prep. These pockets are a portable joy for lunch on the run, whether they are filled with a protein-rich mixture of grilled chicken and tzatziki or a Mediterranean-inspired mix of veggies and hummus.

9. The Charm of Stuffed Avocados: A delicious treat for lunch on-the-go are stuffed avocados, which combine the creamy texture of avocados with a range of delectable fillings. In Skinny Taste Meal Prep, the author examines the allure of packed avocados and provides recipes that highlight the fruit's versatility. These stuffed avocados are a full and convenient lunch choice, whether you fill them with tuna salad, quinoa, or black bean mixtures.

10. Satisfying Soups in Jars: Soups in jars are a new offering from Skinny Taste Meal Prep, catering to people who want a hot, comfortable meal on the go. Layers of ingredients keep these portable soup options fresh until you're ready to eat them. These jarred soups, which range from hot chili to hearty minestrone, are a filling and practical lunchtime option.

You'll learn that lunches don't have to be boring; they can be tasty and portable without compromising on nutrition when you explore the Lunch on the Go chapter of Skinny Taste Meal Prep. Every recipe, which ranges from colorful salads and wraps to inventive roll-ups and filling bowls, is designed to improve your lunchtime experience. Enjoy the satisfaction of eating a tasty, health-conscious dinner that easily fits into your busy schedule as you set off on this culinary adventure. Prepare to change your lunch routine, one tasty and convenient bite at a time.

Chapter 6: Easy-to-Prepare Dinners for Busy Evenings

Dinner is more than simply a meal in the world of Skinny Taste Meal Prep; it's a time to relax, enjoy, and fuel you. We will delve into the art of creating tasty, health-conscious dinners with seven ingredients or less in this chapter, Easy-to-Prepare Dinners for Busy Evenings. Find the delight in preparing healthful evening meals that fit into your busy schedule, from the ease of one-pot miracles to the simplicity of sheet-pan marvels.

6.1 Easy-to-Prepare Dinners for Busy Evenings

1. The Evening Rush: The problem of time limits and the desire for a tasty, home-cooked supper are typically present on busy evenings. Understanding the rigors of contemporary living, Skinny Taste Meal Prep provides a selection of dinner options that are not only flavorful and nutritious, but also simple to make. You may be sure that your evenings will be full of tasty and easy meals thanks to these recipes.

2. Balanced Dinner Solutions: The foundation of a healthy lifestyle is a well-balanced dinner, which gives your body the nourishment it needs to rest and replenish. Dinners from Skinny Taste Meal Prep strike the ideal ratio of whole grains, meats, and veggies, resulting in meals that are filling and nutritious. Encouraging and attainable healthy dinners even on the busiest evenings are the aim.

3. Efficiency in the Kitchen: The secret to Simple Dinners for Busy Evenings is Efficiency. Time-saving methods and simplicity of preparation are the main focus of these recipes. The objective is to expedite the cooking process without sacrificing the meal's quality or flavor, regardless of experience level. Each recipe calls for seven ingredients or less, making them approachable and effective for a stress-free evening.

4. Customization for Variety: Keeping dinner interesting and fun requires variety. Dinners for Skinny Taste Meal Prep provide an open canvas for you to play around with flavors, textures, and ingredients. The recipes are easy to adapt to your own taste preferences and dietary requirements because of their simplicity.

6.2 One-Pot Wonders

1. The Beauty of One-Pot Cooking: In the world of hectic evenings, one-pot marvels are a discovery. The beauty of one-pot cooking, where a single pot becomes the stage for a delectable and hassle-free supper, is celebrated by Skinny Taste Meal Prep. One-pot wonders, which range from robust stews to cozy pastas, reduce cleaning and streamline the cooking process, making them the perfect choice for evenings when time is of the essence.

2. Nourishing Soups and Stews: One-pot marvels that are both warm and nourishing for dinner are soups and stews. The world of filling soups and stews that blend veggies, protein, and tasty broth all in one pot is explored in Skinny Taste Meal Prep, These dishes which range from beef and lentil stew to chicken and vegetable soup, are proof of the rich flavor that can be produced with little work.

3. Effortless Pasta Creations: Pasta recipes are a classic choice for quick and filling meals. Traditional pasta recipes are transformed into simple preparations that can be made in one pot by using Skinny Taste Meal Prep. Whether it's traditional spaghetti bolognese or a penne primavera bursting with vegetables, these one-pot pasta miracles maximize taste without requiring a lot of cooking time.

4. Flavorful Rice and Grain Bowls: Beyond pasta, one-pot miracles include savory grain and rice bowls. Recipes that highlight the adaptability of grains like rice, quinoa, and farro are included in Skinny Taste Meal Prep. These bowls blend grains, veggies, and proteins in one pot for a hearty and filling supper that's simple to make and even more enjoyable to eat.

5. Efficient Stir-Fry Delights: My go-to option for easy and delectable dinners is stir-fried vegetables. With its one-pot recipes, Skinny Taste Meal Prep elevates the efficiency of stir-frying to a whole new level. These tasty stir-fry dishes blend bright veggies, lean proteins, and savory sauces to create an easy dinner that is also a sensory feast.

6. Simmering Casseroles and Bakes: Comfort food is often associated with casseroles and bakes, and Skinny Taste Meal

Prep's one-pot miracles provide that comfort to hectic evenings. These simmering dishes, which range from protein-rich casseroles to cheesy baked pastas, blend layers of ingredients in one dish. The end product is a satisfying and easy supper that requires little work but yields a lot of flavor.

6.3 Sheets-Pan Marvels

1. The Simplicity of Sheet-Pan Cooking: The wonders of sheet pans attest to how easy it is to prepare full dinners with little mess. The technique of sheet-pan cooking, in which a single pan serves as the canvas for a tasty and nourishing dinner, is something that Skinny Taste dinner Prep appreciates. From delicious proteins to roasted vegetables, sheet-pan wonders provide a simple way to produce dinners that are full of flavor and little effort.

2. Roasted Vegetables and More: Roasting is a cooking technique that enhances the inherent flavors of veggies and proteins. With sheet-pan wonders, Skinny Taste Meal Prep delves into the world of roasted veggies and more. These dishes highlight how easy it is to prepare food by just tossing it onto a sheet pan, adding some herbs and spices, and then baking it until it turns golden. These recipes, which range from sheet-pan fajitas to roasted Brussels sprouts, are as colorful and flavorful as they are vibrant.

3. Efficient Protein and Veggie Pairings: The wonders of the sheet pan are adept at matching veggies and proteins in a frugal way. Recipes like balsamic-glazed fish with vibrant bell peppers or lemon herb chicken with roasted asparagus highlight how simple it is to combine protein and vegetables on one sheet pan. As a consequence, you get a balanced supper that needs very little preparation time.

4. Creative One-Pan Dishes: Beyond the ordinary, sheet-pan wonders include inventive one-pan meals that liven up your dinner table. Recipes such as sheet-pan nachos with lean ground turkey, black beans, and cheese or a one-pan chicken with olives and tomatoes with a Mediterranean flair are presented in Skinny Taste Meal Prep. These recipes highlight the variety of tastes and textures that one pan can provide.

5. Effortless Seafood Sheet-Pans: Fans of seafood will love how easy it is to make delicious dinners with seafood sheet pans. Recipes from Skinny Taste Meal Prep highlight the subtle flavors of fish and shellfish and are served with a rainbow of colorful veggies. These recipes, which range from spicy sheet-pan cod with cherry tomatoes to lemon garlic shrimp with roasted broccoli, are easy to make and delicious to consume.

6. Versatile Sheet-Pan Fajitas: Tex-Mex-inspired sheet-pan fajitas are a flexible and well-liked dinner choice that livens up hectic evenings. A range of sheet-pan fajita recipes, including vegetarian options including portobello mushrooms and traditional chicken fajitas, are presented by Skinny Taste Meal Prep. With the help of these recipes, you can make your fajitas with a variety of colorful peppers, onions, and your preferred protein for a tasty and festive supper.

7. Efficiency in Clean-up: The effectiveness of sheet-pan miracles in clean-up is one of their best qualities. These dinners are simple to make and give you more time to unwind and enjoy your evening because there aren't as many pots and pans to clean up afterward. For those looking for a stress-free supper option, sheet-pan cooking's simplicity is revolutionary.

43

You'll learn that dinner doesn't have to sacrifice flavor or nutrition when you explore Skinny Taste Meal Prep's chapter on Easy-to-Prepare Dinners for Busy Evenings. Every recipe is designed to make your evenings stress-free and fulfilling, whether they are sheet-pan miracles or one-pot wonders due to their simplicity or efficiency. As you set out on your culinary adventure, enjoy the satisfaction of making and eating healthful meals that work with your hectic schedule. Prepare to change the way you eat dinner every night, one tasty bite at a time.

Chapter 7: Snack Attack

Snacking isn't an afterthought in the colorful tapestry of Skinny Taste Meal Prep; rather, it's a thoughtfully chosen assortment of Healthy Bites for Anytime Cravings. This chapter takes you on a trip into the realm of guilt-free snacking, where we'll learn how to make tasty, nutritious snacks with just seven ingredients or less. Discover the delight of enjoying snacks that not only tempt your taste senses but also improve your general well-being, from the ease of grab-and-go options to the satisfaction of homemade delicacies.

7.1 Healthy Bites for Anytime Cravings

1. The Craving Conundrum: Anytime a craving arises, Skinny Taste Meal Prep offers Healthy Bites for Anytime Cravings as the perfect way to sate it. This chapter is a celebration of snacks that go beyond mindless snacking, providing a range of choices that will satisfy your palate and feed your body. These snacks, which range from sweet to savory, are made simply and with intention.

2. The Importance of Snacking Mindfully: Mindful snacking is crucial to leading a balanced and healthful lifestyle. The technique of mindful snacking savoring each bite, appreciating the flavors, and selecting snacks that support your nutritional objectives is something that Skinny Taste Meal Prep promotes. You may change snacking from a fleeting indulgence to a conscious and guilt-free activity by approaching it with intention.

3. Balancing Nutrients in Snacks: Nutrient balancing is the key to guilt-free snacking. Proteins, good fats, and carbohydrates are all perfectly balanced in Skinny Taste Meal Prep snacks to provide you long-lasting energy and satisfaction. Whether you're searching for a pre-workout snack or a last-minute afternoon pick-me-up, these recipes make sure that your snacks improve your general health.

4. Snacking for All Occasions: This chapter's snacks are designed to fit a range of events. Skinny Taste Meal Prep provides a variety of options to suit your needs, including on-the-go portability, a sweet treat for a relaxing evening or a crunchy nibble for a movie night. Because these snacks are so flexible, you can select ones that suit your tastes and way of life.

7.2 Guilt-Free Snacking

1. Mindful Choices for Sweet Tooth Cravings: When the urge for something sweet comes, Skinny Taste Meal Prep provides guilt-free snacking options that fulfill without sacrificing health. These tasty sweets are a lovely way to indulge in moderation. They range from fruit and nut combos to energy balls produced with healthy components. The secret is to select guilt-free foods that naturally sweeten due to components like fruits or a small amount of honey.

2. Fruit and Nut Combos: The epitome of guilt-free snacking is the traditional pairing of fruits and nuts. An assortment of fruit and nut combinations that are both filling and healthy are presented in Skinny Taste Meal Prep. These combinations, which include dried apricots with pistachios, banana chips with walnuts, and apple slices with almond butter, offer a variety of tastes and textures for a delightful and healthful snack.

3. Homemade Energy Bars: Energy bars from the store can include a lengthy ingredient list that includes extra sugars and preservatives. Making your own homemade energy bars allows you to be in charge of the ingredients, something that Skinny Taste Meal Prep strongly advocates. Made with a few healthy ingredients (oats, nuts, seeds, and natural sweeteners), these bars are quick and simple to prepare, and they make a filling and practical snack for hectic days.

4. Nutrient-Packed Smoothie Bowls: Smoothie bowls aren't only for breakfast; they also make delicious, guilt-free snacks. Discover the world of nutrient-packed smoothie bowls, which are not only aesthetically pleasing but also a veritable vitamin and mineral powerhouse, in Skinny Taste Meal Prep. For a nutritious and refreshing snack, try these bowls with frozen fruits, leafy greens, and a variety of toppings like nuts and seeds.

5. Crunchy Veggie Sticks and Dips: Enjoying tasty dips with crunchy veggies is a guilt-free and filling snack choice. Recipes from Skinny Taste Meal Prep highlight the crispness of fresh vegetables like bell peppers, carrots, and cucumbers and are served with guacamole, hummus, or Greek yogurt dips. Together, these ingredients provide a filling, low-calorie snack that's ideal for sating appetites in between meals.

6. Smart Popcorn Twists: Popcorn is a popular and adaptable snack that gets a new twist thanks to Skinny Taste Meal Prep's Smart Popcorn Twists. These inventive variations turn popcorn into a tasty and guilt-free snack by air-popping it and adding inventive flavors like nutritional yeast, cinnamon, or a dash of heat. Savor it as a light and filling midday snack or on movie evenings.

7. Protein-Packed Cheese and Nut Platters: Protein-Packed Platters combine cheese and almonds in a filling and healthy dish. A range of cheese and nut combinations are introduced in Skinny Taste Meal Prep, providing a blend of flavors and textures. For a snack high in protein and good fats, try goat cheese with pistachios, sliced cheese with almonds, or a mix of cheeses with walnuts.

8. Frozen Yogurt Bites: Frozen Yogurt Bites are a guilt-free, refreshing dessert from Skinny Taste Meal Prep. Greek yogurt and fresh fruit come together in these bite-sized treats to make a cool, calorie-conscious snack. Add different fruit combinations or a honey drizzle to your frozen yogurt bites to create a sweet and filling treat that's ideal for warm days or anytime cravings.

9. Savory Roasted Chickpeas: Have a taste for something crunchy and savory? Savory Roasted Chickpeas are a new and delicious addition to Skinny Taste Meal Prep. They're also rather healthy. These little morsels become a guilt-free substitute for typical salty snacks by sprinkling chickpeas with a mixture of spices and roasting them until crispy. Savor them by themselves or as a garnish for soups and salads.

10. Dairy-Free Chia Pudding Cups: Chia Pudding Cups are a guilt-free and dairy-free snack option provided by Skinny Taste Meal Prep. These cups turn chia seeds, plant-based milk, and a hint of sweetness into a creamy and filling choice that can be enjoyed anytime. To add taste and texture, personalize your chia pudding by adding toppings like almond butter, fresh berries, or almonds.

11. Mindful Portion Control: It's important to exercise attentive portion management when indulging in guilt-free snacks. The practice of enjoying every bite and paying attention to your body's signals of hunger and fullness is encouraged by Skinny Taste Meal Prep. You can enjoy tasty sweets guilt-free by portioning snacks ahead of time and selecting nutrient-dense selections, which will help you develop a healthy relationship with snacking.

You'll learn that snacking doesn't have to sacrifice taste or nutritional value as you go through Skinny Taste Meal Prep's Snack Attack chapter. Every recipe, from fruit combinations and sweet treats to savory bites and crunchy pleasures, is designed to sate your appetites and improve your general health. As you set out on your gastronomic adventure, savor the delight of nibbling on foods that satisfy your palate and nourish your body. Prepare to change the way you nibble by starting with one tasty and attentive bite.

Chapter 8: Sweet Treats

Explore Desserts without the Guilt on this pleasant trip into Sweet Treats within the delightful world of Skinny Taste Meal Prep. This chapter explores the art of creating delicious treats using seven ingredients or less, and it's a celebration of indulgence done correctly. Discover the delight of indulging in sweets that satiate your palate and support your resolve to Indulge Responsibly, whether they are rich chocolate delights or refreshing fruity treats.

8.1 Desserts without the Guilt

1. A Sweet Affair with Health in Mind: Sweet sweets are meant to be guilt-free in the realm of Skinny Taste Meal Prep, but they frequently straddle the line between indulgence and guilt. This chapter is proof that you may indulge your sweet desire without sacrificing your dedication to leading a healthful lifestyle. The richness of flavors, the delight of textures, and the mindfulness of ingredients come together in desserts without the guilt.

2. Understanding Smart Indulgence: Sweet treats don't always have to be associated with guilt. The philosophy of Smart

Indulgence, in which desserts are prepared with an awareness of portion control, ingredient selection, and nutritional balance, is promoted by Skinny Taste Meal Prep. You can enjoy the sweets in moderation and mindfulness if you choose wisely what to put into your desserts.

3. Balancing Flavors and Nutrients: Desserts without the Guilt find a happy medium between nourishing your body with vital nutrients and sating your sweet tooth. Sweet treats from Skinny Taste Meal Prep are designed to incorporate elements that enhance the dessert's overall nutritional profile, so they're not simply empty calories. Every component, from the sweetness of fruits in their natural state to the richness of nuts, is selected with consideration for both taste and health.

4. Versatility in Dessert Options: This chapter's Sweet Treats are adaptable, satisfying a range of dietary requirements and tastes. Skinny Taste Meal Prep has a variety of dessert options, whether you're a fan of fruity snacks, chocolate, or the ease of no-bake desserts. The intention is to offer options that suit your taste preferences and make it simple to indulge responsibly.

8.2 Indulge Responsibly

1. Portion Control for Pleasure: Controlling your portion sizes is the first step towards responsibly indulging. The concept of enjoying tiny, thoughtfully portioned quantities of sweet sweets is promoted by Skinny Taste Meal Prep. You may completely appreciate the flavors and textures of desserts without going overboard if you prioritize quality over quantity. The secret is to savor every bite and to remember that moderation yields the greatest pleasure.

2. Mindful Ingredient Choices: Making responsible choices regarding the ingredients in your sweets is another way to indulge. Desserts from Skinny Taste Meal Prep put an emphasis on whole, nutrient-dense products while avoiding processed foods, artificial additives, and high sugar content. You can make sweets that not only satiate your appetites but also improve your general health by using ingredients of the highest caliber.

3. Incorporating Nutrient-Rich Elements: Nutrient-rich ingredients can be added to sweet sweets, as Indulge Responsibly explains. Nuts, seeds, and whole grains are examples of ingredients that Skinny Taste Meal Prep promotes using to give desserts more nutrition. These ingredients add vital vitamins and minerals, protein, and good fats to the dish in addition to enhancing its flavor and texture.

4. Embracing Natural Sweeteners: Using natural sweeteners to sweeten sweets is a fundamental component of Indulge Responsibly. In Skinny Taste Meal Prep, substitute sweeteners that give desserts more complexity and richness are examined, including agave nectar, honey, and maple syrup. Accepting the sweetness of foods without overindulging in refined sugars is possible when you utilize natural sweeteners.

5. The Magic of Fresh Fruits: Desserts that emphasize flavor and health tend to have a lot of fresh fruit. The Skinny Taste Meal Prep honors the power of fresh fruits as flavor enhancers and sweeteners. Fresh fruit adds a pleasant and guilt-free treat to sweets, whether it's the natural sweetness of ripe berries, the juiciness of citrus fruits, or the tropical allure of mangoes.

6. Whole Grains for Texture and Nutrients: Sweet sweets made with whole grains have more texture and nutritional richness. In order to give desserts a healthy base, Skinny Taste Meal Prep recommends the use of foods like quinoa, whole wheat flour, and oats. With the addition of fiber, antioxidants, and vital nutrients, these whole grains turn sweets into satisfying delights that also improve general health.

7. The Delight of Dark Chocolate: Rich in flavor and possibly even good for you, dark chocolate is a lovely addition to Skinny Taste Meal Prep sweet delights. The usage of dark chocolate with a high cocoa content, which has less sugar and is full of antioxidants, is examined in Indulge Responsibly. Dark chocolate adds a rich but health-conscious touch to sweets, from chocolate drizzles to rich morsels.

8. Balancing Creaminess with Health: Desserts can have creamy textures without using a lot of fat and heavy cream. Desserts from the Skinny Taste Meal Prep strike a balance between creaminess and health by using items like avocado, Greek yogurt, and coconut milk. These substitutes enhance the luxurious and fulfilling aspect of confections without sacrificing their nutritional worth.

9. Creative Flavors without the Excess: Responsible indulgence enables the investigation of inventive and distinctive taste pairings devoid of surplus carbohydrates and fats. Sweet delights from Skinny Taste Meal Prep offer creative combinations like berries drizzled with balsamic, nuts seasoned with chai, or honey infused with lavender. Desserts become more sophisticated thanks to these inventive tastes, which also make them guilt-free and health-conscious.

10. The Pleasure of No-Bake Options: Skinny Taste Meal Prep provides the delight of No-Bake Options for those times when using the oven seems like too much work. Desserts that may be prepared without baking are included in Indulge Responsibly, offering a simple and quick approach to sate your sweet tooth. These sweets, which range from chilled fruit tarts to no-bake energy bites, prove that decadence can be both tasty and simple.

You'll learn that, when prepared with intention, desserts can be decadent and guilt-free as you delve into Skinny Taste Meal Prep's Sweet Treats chapter. Every recipe is an ode to responsible indulgence, showcasing everything from the richness of dark chocolate to the freshness of fruits and the inventiveness of flavor combinations. Savor the delight of sweet delicacies as you set off on this gastronomic adventure; they will not only satisfy your palate but also reinforce your resolve to lead a balanced and healthful lifestyle. Prepare to change the way you enjoy dessert, one delicious taste at a time.

Chapter 9: Meal Prep Plans

In the disciplined realm of Skinny Taste Meal Prep, batch cooking techniques and weekly meal prep schedule creation combine efficiency and flavor. This chapter will show you how to turn your kitchen into a center of efficiency and well-thought-out design. Savor the satisfaction of cooking healthful, flavorful meals with just seven items or less, all while saving time and money for a week full of excellent meals.

9.1 Weekly Meal Prep Schedules

1. The Foundation of Success: Meal preparation is more than just a habit; it's the cornerstone to successfully upholding a balanced, healthful lifestyle. Weekly Meal Prep Schedules are the cornerstone of effective and mindful eating in the context of Skinny Taste Meal Prep. This section offers a meal plan template so you can make sure you always have a range of delicious options available to you throughout the week.

2. Planning for Nutritional Balance: Planning for nutritional balance is essential to successful meal prep. Weekly meal prep schedules that incorporate a range of proteins, veggies, whole grains, and healthy fats are encouraged by Skinny Taste Meal Prep. You can guarantee that your body gets the vital nutrients it requires to flourish by planning your meals carefully, which will support long-term vitality and general wellbeing.

3. Streamlining the Shopping Process: Weekly Meal Prep Schedules are made to make grocery shopping more efficient. Efficiency starts at the supermarket. You may create well-organized shopping lists based on your weekly food plan with the help of Skinny Taste food Prep. You may make the most of your time and resources by concentrating on using fresh and whole products, so you'll have everything you need to execute your meal prep plan.

4. Balancing Variety and Simplicity: Because diversity is the flavor of life, Skinny Taste Meal Prep stresses the value of striking a balance between complexity and variation in your weekly meal prep plans. You may prevent boredom and maintain the excitement of your meals by combining a variety of flavors and components. However, the ease of use that comes with utilizing seven ingredients or fewer every recipe guarantees that meal prep stays manageable and effective.

5. The Time-Saving Magic of Prep: Meal prep involves more than just cooking; it also involves arranging supplies to maximize time savings during the week. By adding prep-ahead techniques into your weekly meal prep schedules, Skinny Taste Meal Prep brings time-saving magic into your routine. These preparation actions, which range from slicing vegetables to marinating proteins, facilitate speedy meal assembly, particularly on hectic days.

6. Portion Control for Success: A key component of weekly meal prep schedules that helps you succeed in keeping up a healthy lifestyle is portion control. During the meal prep process, Skinny Taste Meal Prep encourages thoughtful portioning to make sure that each dish is in line with your nutritional objectives. You can practice mindful eating and save time over the week by separating meals into smaller portions.

7. Creating a Balanced Meal Calendar: At the core of Weekly

Meal Prep Schedules is a thoughtful meal calendar. Using Skinny Taste Meal Prep, you can create a well-balanced meal plan that takes into account your weekly schedule, dietary requirements, and personal preferences. Every day is a culinary adventure that advances your general well-being and appreciation of food, from filling meals to transportable lunches and easy snacks.

8. Flexibility for Real Life: Skinny Taste Meal Prep recognizes the value of flexibility in weekly meal prep schedules, even if structure is still important. Because life is dynamic, unforeseen things can happen. This chapter delves into tactics for modifying your meal plan to suit alterations in your calendar, guaranteeing that meal preparation stays an instrument for accomplishment rather than a cause of anxiety.

9.2 Batch Cooking Strategies

1. Efficiency in the Kitchen: The key to effective meal prep is batch cooking, which Skinny Taste Meal Prep reveals as well as the techniques for becoming an expert in it. With the help of batch cooking strategies, you may produce big quantities of essential components that can be used to create a variety of meals throughout the week. These strategies are intended to maximize efficiency in the kitchen. This section contains instructions on how to turn your kitchen into an extremely productive space.

2. Identifying Key Ingredients: The first step in batch cooking is to determine the essential elements that serve as the basis for several meals. According to Skinny Taste Meal Prep, grains like quinoa and rice, proteins like chicken, beans, and tofu, and roasted veggies are essential components of batch cooking strategies. You may easily create a variety of meals with little effort by prepping these ingredients in bulk.

3. Cooking in Batches for Variety: Eating the same dinner every day is not the result of batch cooking. The idea of Cooking in Batches for Variety, wherein staple components are turned into several meals throughout the week, is introduced in Skinny Taste Meal Prep. To make sure your meals are always interesting and varied, try putting some grilled chicken on top of salads, wraps, and stir-fries.

3. Storage Solutions for Freshness: For meal prep to be successful, foods that have been batch-cooked must be kept fresh. In Skinny Taste Meal Prep, storage options that maintain the textures and aromas of prepared foods are examined. These tips, which range from freezer-friendly packaging to airtight containers, guarantee that your batch-cooked foods stay tasty and accessible whenever you need them.

4. Strategic Reheating Techniques: Reheating is an essential component of Batch Cooking Strategies. To preserve the quality of your prepared meals, Skinny Taste Meal Prep offers thoughtful reheating methods. These techniques, which range from crisping food in the oven to steaming grains to reheat them, guarantee that your meals taste as good as they did when they were newly made.

5. Creating Modular Meals: The foundation of batch cooking strategies is modular meals. You can create modular components that can be combined and rearranged to create a variety of meals with the help of Skinny Taste Meal Prep. A batch of roasted veggies, for instance, may be mixed and matched with various proteins and grains over the course of the week, creating countless dinner options without requiring a lot of cooking every day.

6. Integrating Sauces and Dressings: The flavor enhancers that transform batch-cooked goods into delicious dinners are sauces and dressings. The idea of incorporating sauces and dressings into your batch cooking strategies is presented in Skinny Taste Meal Prep. You don't have to do complex cooking every day of the week to add a pop of flavor to your meals by prepping adaptable sauces.

7. Repurposing Leftovers Creatively: Batch Cooking Strategies are inventive ways to repurpose leftovers beyond just reheating them. The skill of creating novel and interesting meals out of leftovers is explored in Skinny Taste Meal Prep. Showcasing the creativity that comes with bulk cooking, roasted veggies from dinner can be used as a tasty addition to a grain bowl for lunch or an omelet in the morning.

8. Weekend Batch Cooking Rituals: A key component of effective weekly meal prep schedules is developing a ritual for batch cooking on the weekends. Skinny Taste Meal Prep walks you through the process of organizing weekend bulk cooking into a methodical and effective routine. By dedicating specific time for tasks like slicing vegetables, marinating proteins, or making sauces, you can make your kitchen a center of efficiency.

9. Celebrating Seasonal and Fresh Ingredients: Batch Cooking Strategies emphasize efficiency, whereas Skinny Taste Meal Prep highlights the value of savoring fresh, in-season ingredients. Your meals take on a dynamic flavor and nutritious variety when you use the best that each season has to offer. This chapter helps you create a farm-to-table experience by coordinating your batch cooking with seasonal ingredients.

10. Scaling Strategies for Busy Weeks: It could be necessary to scale up batch cooking strategies and do more preparation during busy weeks. How to scale your batch cooking efforts to meet the demands of a busy schedule is covered in Skinny Taste Meal Prep. These scaling techniques, which range from doubling recipes to making bigger batches of essential components, guarantee that your kitchen is well-stocked during periods of higher activity.

You'll discover the keys to effective and health-conscious meal planning as you delve into the Meal Prep Plans chapter of Skinny Taste Meal Prep. Every component of meal prep is designed to make it a smooth and pleasurable part of your routine, from planning weekly meal prep schedules that strike a balance between diversity and simplicity to becoming proficient in batch cooking strategies that turn your kitchen into a space of productivity. Prepare to transform your cooking style one well-planned and delectable dinner at a time.

Chapter 10: Success Stories

Success stories are the colorful threads that tell the touching tales of real-life transformations and victories in Skinny Taste Meal Prep. This chapter celebrates the travels travelled, the challenges faced, and the significant effects that nutritious dishes with seven ingredients or less can have on people's lives. Learn about the motivation and inspiration behind amazing transformations and the creation of a sense of success within the Skinny Taste community through their testimonies.

10.1 Real-Life Transformations

1. The Power of Personal Stories: Real-life makeovers include a whole change in lifestyle, perspective, and overall wellbeing in addition to physical adjustments. Skinny Taste Meal Prep acknowledges that every journey is distinct and important and embraces the Power of Personal Stories. This part explores the personal accounts of people who have adopted the concepts outlined in the cookbook, sharing their experiences of inner and outer transformation.

2. From Challenges to Triumphs: The success stories of Skinny Taste Meal Prep are no different from the obstacles that precede any transformation. People talk about how they overcame obstacles, whether it was dealing with hectic schedules, unsure culinary choices, or health issues. For anyone who might be facing comparable challenges on their own path to a better and more satisfying life, these tales provide hope.

3. Embracing Healthy Habits: Adopting healthy recipes requires more than just cleaning the plate; it also entails developing good habits. In Skinny Taste Meal Prep, the authors examine how readers have adopted Healthy Habits as a consequence of incorporating the cookbook's ideas into their daily routines. These practices, which range from mindful eating to regular meal planning, serve as the cornerstone for long-term success and wellbeing.

4. Achieving Balance: Finding balance is an important accomplishment in a society where we are frequently pulled in many directions. Success stories from Skinny Taste Meal Prep show how people have achieved life balance by putting their health first without compromising taste or enjoyment. These stories highlight the healing potential of preparing meals that recognize the body's need for joy and fulfillment in each mouthful.

5. Enhanced Energy and Vitality: A recurring theme in success tales is feeling more alive and energetic. Skinny Taste Meal Prep has emerged as a major force behind those who want to shed pounds but also feel more energised and alive. By sharing healthy recipes and thoughtful meal preparation, people talk about how they've regained their enthusiasm for life and are now welcoming each day with renewed energy.

6. Culinary Confidence: For many people, the desire to become more confident in their cooking abilities and learn culinary skills is the first step towards embracing healthier recipes. Success stories from Skinny Taste Meal Prep explore how people who were once afraid to cook have grown into self-assured culinary enthusiasts. The cookbook's focus on using only seven ingredients or less and simplicity provides a solid base for developing one's creative and culinary skills.

7. Positive Body Image: The path to health cannot be separated from the development of a positive body image. Success stories from Skinny Taste Meal Prep highlight the significant influence that embracing healthy meals has on one's sense of self and acceptance of their body. These tales illustrate the necessity of nurturing the spirit in addition to the body by showing the transformational path from self-judgment to self-love.

8. Inspiring Others: Within the Skinny Taste community, success stories frequently go beyond individual accomplishments to serve as sources of motivation for others. People talk about how their health journeys have encouraged friends, family, and even entire communities to start their own health journeys. These tales highlight the possibility for communal well-being and the beneficial spill over effect of positive change.

10.2 Testimonials from the Skinny Taste Community

1. The Collective Voice: Skinny Taste community testimonials serve to magnify the voices of those who have adopted the cookbook's guiding principles. This section is a patchwork of personal accounts, endorsements, and sincere observations that demonstrate how Skinny Taste Meal Prep has impacted a variety of lifestyles.

2. Community Support and Connection: The Skinny Taste community is more than just a group of people; it's a source of connection and support. Testimonials show how important a part the community has played in helping one another on their journeys. Through social media groups, online forums, or local meet-ups, people exchange the spirit of support and friendship that has grown to be an essential aspect of the Skinny Taste experience.

3. Celebrating Diversity in Journeys: Testimonials highlight the Diversity in trips within the Skinny Taste community, as no two trips are alike. The cookbook's tenets have found resonance with a wide range of demands and objectives, from those looking to lose weight to those managing certain health concerns or just trying to improve their general well-being. These testimonies highlight Skinny Taste Meal Prep's adaptability and inclusion.

4. Family and Community Bonding: Skinny Taste Meal Prep has an impact on community and family bonding in addition to the individual. Testimonials show how families and communities are now working together to embrace healthier cuisine. Relationships become stronger and more cohesive when people cook together, share meals, and encourage one another's aspirations.

5. Rediscovering the Joy of Cooking: Testimonials express the happiness that results from rediscovering cooking as a delight. Many people tell us how the cookbook has made them fall in love again with cooking, turning what they always thought of as a duty into a fun and rewarding hobby. With its approachable dishes and inventive simplicity, Skinny Taste Meal Prep turns into a joyful cooking adventure.

6. Inspirational Meal Prep Rituals: In the Skinny Taste group, meal preparation evolves into a series of Inspiring Meal Prep Rituals. Testimonials reveal how people have included meal prep into their weekly routines, enjoying the process of preparing, cooking, and indulging in wholesome, delectable meals. These customs develop into deliberate feeding and self-care times.

7. Culinary Creativity Unleashed: Lean Taste Meal Prep is a platform for Unleashed Culinary Creativity. Testimonials show how people have used the recipes in the booklet as a jumping off point for their own culinary adventures. Whether it's customizing flavors or creating new recipes based on the ideas of minimalism, the cookbook serves as a spark for culinary creativity.

8. Sustainable and Long-Term Change: The ability to bring about long-lasting, sustainable change is the real test of success. Testimonials from the Skinny Taste community highlight how embracing healthier cuisine has evolved from a transient project to a way of life. People describe how the cookbook's ideas have permeated every aspect of their everyday lives, producing long-term health advantages and a steady sense of wellbeing.

9. Empowerment through Nutrition: The subject of Empowerment through Nutrition is reinforced by testimonies. People talk about how knowing how food affects their bodies has given them the ability to make deliberate and well-informed decisions. By empowering people to take charge of their health, creating a sense of agency, and laying the groundwork for a healthier future, Skinny Taste Meal Prep becomes an invaluable tool.

10. A Heartfelt Thank You: After reading through the testimonies, the Skinny Taste community extends a sincere thank you to all of the creators, contributors, and other members who have helped them on their transforming journeys. Gratitude is expressed in these remarks, creating a chorus of appreciation for the beneficial effects of Skinny Taste Meal Prep on people's life and the community as a whole.

You will see first-hand the transformative effect of healthy foods made with seven ingredients or less as you go through the Success Stories chapter of Skinny Taste Meal Prep. Each narrative, which ranges from touching testimonies to real-life makeovers, demonstrates how the cookbook can uplift, encourage, and foster a feeling of community. Prepare to be inspired, driven, and uplifted as you join the group on its path to a happier, healthier life one success story at a time.

Chapter 11: Conclusion

We've explored the domains of health, flavor, and simplicity in The Skinny Taste Meal Prep, learning how to create delicious recipes with just seven ingredients or less. As our culinary journey draws to a close, let's take time to celebrate our victories, look back on the voyage, and prepare for the next phase of our journey a lifetime of happiness and health.

11.1 Final Thoughts on Healthy Meal Prep

The Simplicity Advantage: The Simplicity Advantage is the beating heart of Skinny Taste Meal Prep. Simplicity is a need in the fast-paced world of modern living, not merely a preference. The cookbook's commitment to seven-ingredient recipes isn't about constraint; rather, it's about freedom. It's an invitation to appreciate the elegance of simple cooking, in which each dish is a celebration of flavor and easiness and every item has a purpose.

Flavorful Simplicity: Concluding Remarks on Healthful Meal Planning emphasize the important fact that flavor need not be sacrificed for simplicity. It is evident from the rich tapestry of dishes at Skinny Taste Meal Prep that less really may be more when it comes to flavor, vibrancy, and satisfaction. The cookbook dispels the myth that eating healthily has to mean dull food by demonstrating how a few well-selected components can take meals to entirely new levels of flavor and delight.

Mindful Nourishment: In the context of healthy meal prep, nourishment transcends the physical and takes on the form of an intentional activity. Concluding Remarks: Mindful Nourishment explores the idea that each meal is a chance to respect the body and spirit. Skinny Taste Meal Prep invites people to enjoy the process of creating meals, taste every bite, and embrace the happiness that comes from feeding oneself purposefully and with intention.

The Wellness Symphony: Ultimately, Healthy Meal Prep presents a vision of a Wellness Symphony in which every recipe plays a part in creating a harmonic whole of a balanced and healthful lifestyle. It's not about isolated spurts of self-control but rather an ongoing stream of healthy decisions that combine to create a harmonious whole. Through regular meals and routines,

Skinny Taste Meal Prep becomes a conductor, assisting people in creating a symphony of health.

Efficiency in Action: Healthy meal prep's efficiency is a type of self-care, not just a time-saving tactic. Final Thoughts examine how time may be regained, stress can be decreased, and a sense of control can be fostered through efficiency in the kitchen. With Skinny Taste Meal Prep, preparing meals is no longer a chore but a productive habit that lets people spend their time on the things that really count.

Culinary Empowerment: Concluding Remarks on Healthful Meal Planning embrace the feeling of Culinary Empowerment that results from learning how to cook simply and healthfully. The cookbook turns into a guide, enabling people to confidently traverse the kitchen, try out different flavors, and modify recipes to their own preferences. Beyond the kitchen, culinary empowerment influences decisions that affect one's general well-being.

Balancing Act: A key concept in the quest for health is balance. Concluding Remarks highlight the need of striking a balance between providing the body with nourishment and relishing the joys of food. The philosophy behind Skinny Taste Meal Prep is to help people achieve balance in their diets by allowing them to savor a range of flavors and textures while making sure that every mouthful meets their nutritional needs.

Building Healthy Habits: Healthy meal preparation is an ongoing process that offers the chance to establish the groundwork for developing healthy habits. Concluding Remarks explore the idea of habit formation, in which routines that are shaped by the cookbook become second nature. These practices mindful eating, meal planning on a weekly basis, or experimenting in the kitchen become the cornerstones of long-term wellbeing.

A Celebration of Food: The Skinny Taste Meal Prep is fundamentally a celebration of food. Concluding Remarks are in line with the delight that arises from realizing the variety of tastes, the depth of flavor, and the skill involved in preparing meals. The cookbook encourages people to enjoy the process of creating wholesome and delectable food as well as the act of eating.

11.2 Continuing the Journey

- **A Culinary Odyssey:** Even if The Skinny Taste Meal Prep is coming to an end, the experience continues it just gets better. Continuing the Journey extends an invitation to live a simple, flavorful, and health-conscious lifestyle. It's a dedication to extending the concepts of nutritious food preparation into the future and expanding upon the framework established by the cookbook.

- **Integrating New Discoveries:** Continuing the Journey is an ever-changing process of development and learning. Individuals get the chance to investigate and incorporate New Discoveries as they grow more acquainted with the fundamentals of Skinny Taste Meal Prep. This chapter fosters an attitude of culinary exploration and advancement through activities including customizing recipes, attempting novel ingredients, and experimenting with creative cooking methods.

- **Culinary Creativity Unleashed:** Culinary Creativity Unleashed is augmented by Skinny Taste Meal Prep. Taking the base of simplicity and adding creative flair to it is part of continuing the journey. It's a chance to add unique touches, play around with flavors, and create new recipes based on the ideas in the cookbook. The kitchen serves as a creative and expressive blank canvas.

- **Seasonal and Local Exploration:** Investigating locally and seasonally produced foods is part of continuing the journey. By learning to listen to the cycles of the natural world, people can prepare their meals in accordance with the seasons, savoring the bounty and freshness that each one offers. This investigation links people to the local food scene while also bringing diversity to meals.

- **Expanding the Culinary Repertoire:** Extending the Culinary Repertoire is the next step in the trip. Although Skinny Taste Meal Prep offers a wide variety of dishes, there's always space for experimentation and variety. People can experiment with different cooking methods, draw inspiration from a variety of cuisines, and progressively broaden their culinary repertoire to incorporate a wider range of flavors and techniques.

- **Sharing the Joy:** Sharing the Joy of preparing nutritious meals with others is part of carrying on the Journey. The joy of the kitchen becomes a shared experience, whether it's showing friends and family tasty, health-conscious recipes or giving back to the larger Skinny Taste community. Through encouraging others to set out on their own journeys, people make a communal contribution to the celebration of health and wellbeing.

- **Mindful Eating as a Lifestyle**: Eating mindfully becomes a lifestyle rather than just a technique. A crucial component of carrying on the Journey is incorporating mindful eating into everyday activities. It's about developing a strong bond with the process of eating and enjoying every meal for what it is nourishing food. Beyond the kitchen, mindful eating affects decisions and perspectives about food in many facets of life.

- **Building a Legacy of Health:** The path assumes a profound dimension when people concentrate on leaving a legacy of health. Carrying on the Journey turns into a legacy-building project that affects not only one's own well-being but also the health and lifestyle choices of coming generations. Individuals contribute to a long-lasting legacy of wellbeing and energy by establishing the fundamentals of good meal preparation.

- **Evolving Wellness Rituals:** Well-being is a dynamic state that changes with experience and time. Adapting Wellness Rituals to new situations and requirements is part of continuing the journey. The process becomes an engaging and unique investigation of what it means to live a long and healthy life, whether it involves modifying food patterns to fit various life stages or adding new wellness routines.

- **Gratitude for the Journey:** A sense of thankfulness for the journey emerges as a compass for those who choose to continue the Journey. An appreciation for the flavors encountered, the knowledge gained, and the changes accomplished lend a sense of gratitude to the continuing journey. The voyage turns into an ongoing celebration of the happiness that comes from taking care of one's body and spirit.

As we come to the end of The Skinny Taste Meal Prep: Healthy Recipes with 7 Ingredients or less, we start a new chapter in our never-ending exploration of flavor, health, and wellbeing. May your journey be full of gastronomic joys, life-changing experiences, and a legacy of health that stretches far into the future as you incorporate the concepts of flavor, simplicity, and health-conscious cooking into your daily life. Salutations, and May the happiness that comes with leading a healthy lifestyle journey with you.

About the Author

Dr. Adam C. stands as a beacon of inspiration in the fields of medicine, nutrition, and self-help, with a remarkable journey that exemplifies the transformative power of healthy living. Armed with a professional master's degree in health nutrition and years of experience, Dr. C. has become a guiding light for individuals seeking to embrace vibrant well-being and lead happier lives.

From an early age, Dr. C. navigated through a myriad of health challenges that ranged from genetic predispositions to the pitfalls of unhealthy eating. His personal struggle ignited a flame of determination within him, one that was fueled by the belief that the human body possesses an incredible ability to heal and rejuvenate through the right nourishment. Through steadfast dedication, Dr. C. managed to conquer his own ailments and emerged as a living testament to the transformative potential of a well-balanced lifestyle.

What sets Dr. Adam C. apart is his rich tapestry of experiences, having been deeply immersed in groundbreaking research in health food and diet-related domains. His quest to uncover the hidden treasures of nutrients within our meals has led to groundbreaking revel actions that empower individuals to extract the maximum benefit from their dietary choices. Dr. C.'s research has not only contributed to the scientific community but has also served as a roadmap for countless individuals striving to optimize their health.

However, it is not just Dr. C.'s academic prowess that has touched lives it is his unparalleled compassion and empathy that truly make him a beacon of hope. His personal journey of triumph over adversity infuses his guidance with an authentic understanding of the challenges his readers and patients face. Dr. C. doesn't just prescribe nutritional plans; he fosters a deep connection with his audience, instilling in them the confidence to embark on their own transformative journeys.

Dr. Adam C.'s holistic approach reaches beyond the confines of traditional medicine. His insights have translated into self-help resources that empower individuals to take charge of their wellness narrative. His words resonate on paper as they do in person, making his books not mere guides, but trusted companions on the path to vitality.

In the realm of health and nutrition, Dr. C. shines as a true luminary. His core strengths lie in his ability to synthesize complex scientific findings into practical, actionable advice that individuals from all walks of life can seamlessly integrate into their routines. Dr. C.'s legacy is not just a collection of breakthroughs; it is a testament to the extraordinary potential that lies within each of us to overcome obstacles and embrace a life brimming with health, happiness, and fulfillment.

As an experienced doctor, passionate nutritionist, and empathetic author, Dr. Adam C. continues to transform lives, showing us that the journey to a healthier, happier existence is within our grasp, waiting to be unlocked through the power of informed choices and unwavering determination.